Lose weight fast for women

Inhalt

According to data from some WHO global estimates in 2016, about 1.9 billion people representing more than 39% of adults aged 18 years and above were overweight. Of this percentage, 40% were women. According to these same estimates, global overweight problems have nearly tripled since 1975. Once considered a high-income country problem, overweight is now on the rise in low and middle-income countries, particularly in urban settings. In 2014, the proportion of women in the EU considered as being overweight or obese fell with increasing education level. Contrary to what some may believe, it is not the US that tops the chart, but rather American Samoa where a whopping 74.6 percent are considered to be obese. A slew of other South Pacific nations follow, including Nauru, Tonga, Samoa,

Palau and Kiribati. Kuwait is the only country outside the region to feature in the top 10.

1.1   Factors that contribute to overweight

People develop overweight when their body stores more calories than it uses over time. Your body needs calories (and essential vitamins, minerals, and other nutrients) to work properly and to be active. But if your body stores more calories than it uses, you will gain weight. This is primarily caused by poor dietary choices. Aside accumulation of excess calories, there are also a number of factors that can play a role in weight gain.

These include:

- **Genes and family background**: Overweight tends to run in families. But there is not one "fat" gene. There are many genes that may combine to increase your likelihood of becoming overweight. The situation you live in also affects your genes. When you are a baby or young child, your parents or caregivers control your eating and physical activity. This family background can contribute to your susceptibility to weight gain.

- **Metabolism**: Your metabolism rates (how fast your body "burns" calories) may vary for a lot of reasons, and this can influence your weight. For instance, you're expected to burn calories slower as a woman compared to a man because men usually have more muscles and less fat than women do. A woman's metabolism may change throughout her life, such as with the hormonal changes that happen during puberty, pregnancy, and menopause.

- **Pregnancy effects**: During Pregnancy, a woman gains weight and more body fat. In addition, it's often difficult for a new mother to find the time to exercise and sleep. And she'll need both to shed those extra pounds. However, breastfeeding does help with burning calories and weight loss at this stage of life.

- **Menopause**: Women also tend to accumulate fat in their abdomen during menopause. This is usually due to a loss of hormones and a slower metabolism. Some women even have a name for their new pot belly — meno-pot.

- **Environment:** Your environment largely influences your ability to maintain a healthy weight. If you live in a place where there are not enough parks, sidewalks, or affordable gyms, you may find it hard to stay physically active and shed excess calories in your body. There's also the problem of access to supermarkets that sell affordable healthy foods, such as fresh fruits and vegetables.

- **PCOS struggles**: As much as 10% of women across the globe are known to suffer from polycystic ovary syndrome (PCOS). This condition is characterized by a hormonal imbalance that makes weight loss more difficult and causes menstrual irregularity.

- **Health Conditions and Medications:** Some hormonal problems such as underactive thyroid, Cushing syndrome and Polycystic Ovary Syndrome (POCS) are known to cause overweight. Certain medications like some corticosteroids, antidepressants and diabetes medicines may also increase your likelihood of putting on excess weight by reducing metabolic rate or increasing appetite.

- **Age:** As you age, you lose muscle. And with less muscle to burn calories, you will need fewer calories, thus slowing down your metabolism.

1.2 How do I know if I have overweight or obesity?

The Body Mass Index (BMI) is the universally acceptable method for finding out whether your weight is in a healthy or unhealthy range.

BMI = your weight (kg) / your height (metres).

The tool is primarily used to estimate

body fat. BMI gives you a good idea of how healthy your weight is. Generally, a BMI of 25kg/m^2 to 29.9kg/m^2 is considered to be overweight while a BMI of 30kg/m^2 is considered to be obese. However, BMI doesn't tell the whole story and can be typically less accurate in some people than in others. For example, if you are very muscular, you may be healthy even if your BMI is above 25. This is because muscle weighs more than fat.

Another method to figure out if you have a healthy weight is to measure your waist circumference (the distance around your waist). Waist circumference is measured and categorized into desirable, high and very high, by sex-specific threshold:

- Men: Desirable = Less than 94, High = 94-102, Very high = More than 102

- Women: Desirable = Less than 80, High = 80-88, Very high = More than 88

It is generally acceptable among researchers and doctors that women with a waist circumference larger than 35 inches are at higher risk for many health problems caused by overweight or obesity.

1.3 Does overweight affect some women more than others?

Women of all ages, races, and ethnicities are susceptible to overweight issues. But overweight issues are notoriously prevalent among some groups:

- About 4 in 5 black or African-American women have overweight or obesity.

- More than 3 in 4 Hispanic or Latina women have overweight or obesity.

- Lesbians and bisexual women are more likely to have overweight or obesity than heterosexual women.

Overweight may increase your susceptibility to many health problems such as:

- Type 2 diabetes
- High blood pressure
- Heart disease and strokes
- Certain types of cancer
- Sleep apnea
- Osteoarthritis
- Fatty liver disease
- Kidney disease
- Increase risk for caesarean delivery (C-section)
-

Want to know how to lose weight fast? While there are so many appealing weight-loss plans out there, it is important that you consider the right option for you before embarking on anyone. The trick is, if you're aiming to lose a lot of weight (> 15lbs) then a longer-term diet might be better for you. But if you're interested in diet plans that will deliver weight-loss results fast, below is a comprehensive list of quick fix diet plans that work. In fact, if done well, you could lose up to 10lbs in just seven days! Just take a look at how each work and choose the one you want to get started with.

➢

✓ **How it works**

The 5:2 diet is a type of fasting involving eating about 25% of recommended calorie needs (about 500-600 calories) on two scheduled fasting days and then eating normally the other five days that week. However, 5:2 diet plan founder Dr Michael Mosely has also said that dieters can eat up to 800 calories on fast days and achieve the same results. According to new research people who follow a 5:2 diet plan lose weight quicker and in a healthier way to other diets. UK researchers discovered that 5:2 dieters achieved a five per cent weight loss within two months and had lower blood pressure.

✓ **How much weight can I lose?**

You can lose up to 5 per cent of your weight in fewer than 60 days.

✓ **Pros**

- Proven health benefits

- No foods are off-limits

- You get to choose your fasting days

- Sustainable once in the habit

✓ **Cons**

- Difficult to start

- Possibility of over-eating

- Severe side effects including hunger, fatigue, weakness,

headaches, irritability, mood swings, and difficulty falling sleep.

- Not ideal for everyone especially pregnant women, those who have type 1 diabetes, hypoglycaemia or fertility issues.

✓ **How it works**

The nut and muesli diet involves eating plenty of nuts and muesli. Slimmers normally avoid nuts like the plague as they're so high in calories. But, eaten in the right way, they could be handy when it comes to battling the bulge, according to natural health expert Michael van Straten. He has devised this week-long diet which uses nuts and muesli to help you lose up to half a stone while still providing your body with everything it needs. Muesli, especially, will keep you feeling fuller for longer and so help you avoid dangerous cravings for sweet things.

✓ **How much weight can I lose?**

You can lose up to 7lbs in 7 days.

✓ **Pros**

- Rich in fibre

- Good for diabetics

- Keeps you energetic

- Controls blood pressure

- Full of antioxidants

- Boost immunity

  ✓ **Cons**

- Not balanced enough to replace all of your other meals

- Will not change the eating habits that put the weight on in the first place, and almost guarantees that you will put it all back on the minute you stop the diet

  ✓ **How it works**

Slimfast is a meal replacement plan that allows you to eat up to six times a day. With the Slimfast plan, you eat two Slimfast meal replacements, three 100-calorie snacks (Slimfast snack bars, fruits, veggies, or even nuts), and one 500-calorie meal that you provide. Its most famous products are the milkshake-style drinks that you have instead of breakfast and lunch.

✓ **How much weight can I lose?**

Slimfast MD Brunilda Nazario claims you can lose up to 7lb during the first week and a steady 1lb a week after that.

✓ **Pros**

- Easily accessible
- Less expensive than other commercial plans
- Easy to follow

- Portion controlled

  ✓ **Cons**

- Heavily processed food

- Does not teach healthy eating skills, like portion control, calorie counting, or low-calorie cooking

- No face-to-face support

- Taste

➤ Juice diets

  ✓ **How it works**

There are lots of different juice diets around but they are all based on the same idea – consuming a variety of juiced fruits and vegetables. Many juice diets involve abstaining from eating other foods and only drinking juice, while some involve eating particular solid foods as well. The most extreme juice diets are typically restricted to a short period of time – often between 3-7 days.

✓ How much weight can I lose?

You can lose up to 7lbs in 7 days.

✓ Pros

- High in vitamins and minerals
- Rich in anti-inflammatory compounds that may boost the immune system
- Remove toxins from the body
- Can help improve digestion by introducing healthy enzymes that make the gut work more efficiently

✓ Cons

- Large quantities may be harmful to those with kidney disorders.

- If a person consumes juices that are unpasteurized or have not had another treatment to remove bacteria, they are at greater risk of illness.

- If the juice contains laxatives or other methods of bowel stimulation, a person can lose too many nutrients in their stool. This can cause dehydration and imbalanced electrolytes.

- Consuming juices with an insufficient number of calories can lead to symptoms such as fainting, weakness, headache, etc, relating to low blood sugar because the body is deprived of enough energy.

- Risk of kidney damage.

> ➢ Cabbage Soup Diet

> ✓ **How it works**

The Cabbage Soup Diet is an extremely low-fat, high fibre diet that lasts seven days. The diet works exactly as its name implies – for one week, you eat almost nothing but homemade cabbage soup. Each day, you can also have 1-2 other foods, such as skim milk, fruits or vegetables. It's only designed as a kick-start to help you lose weight quickly and is not supposed to be a long-term healthy eating plan. The Cabbage Soup diet is also known by other names, such as the Sacred Heart Hospital Diet or the Mayo Clinic Diet.

✓ **How much weight can I lose?**

You can lose up to 10lbs in 7 days.

✓ **Pros**

- You are not forced to go hungry, as you may eat as you want each day

- It is fairly easy to follow, with simple rules that take the guesswork out of dieting

- It is affordable as you're only buying cabbage, vegetables and a little meat.

- Encourages the intake of a whole range of fruit and vegetables, thus increasing the intake of fibre. High fibre can help you manage your blood cholesterol, which reduces your risk of cardiovascular disease.

✓ **Cons**

- The diet is deficient in many vitamins and minerals and offers no real source of protein on most days.
- The diet is bland, making it hard to endure for an entire week
- Meals are low in calories and may be difficult to reach 1,200 calories

per day recommended minimum to maintain a stable weight for women

- May cause flatulence and cramping due to high fibre contents

- May cause gallbladder issues

  ➢ **The Fast and Easy Diet**

    ✓ **How it works**

This simple meal planner will help you shop and prepare for your 1,200 calorie-a-day diet. It encourages you to eat slowly, have protein in very meal and make sensible food swaps.

    ✓ **How much weight can I lose?**

Proponents of the plan says you can lose as much as 4lbs in 7 days

➢ **Lose a Pound a Day Diet**

✓ **How it works**

Developed by Rocco DiSpirito, renowned award winning chef, this month-long plan starts with a seven-day detox and then three weeks 'maintenance'. The diet is basically a low calorie, low carb and high protein diet program. Over the whole month you could lose up to a stone. The meal planner is based on the diet of the Swiss, as they are officially the slimmest people in Europe. The diet also gives you simple shopping list rules of what to buy and what to avoid.

✓ **How much weight can I lose?**

You can lose as much as 7lbs in 7 days.

✓ **Pros**

- Flushes harmful toxins out from your body

- Specifically selected foods of the program will stimulate growth of good bacteria in your body which further will work towards your total well-being

- Foods such as yogurt, grapefruit, etc are given great emphasis by the diet program. These foods will rejuvenate your body and skin and will make you look younger and healthier

- You will get rid of high blood pressure and high sugar level while following the diet program

  ✓ **Cons**

- Side effects including headaches, irritability, fatigue, dizziness, menstrual irregularities, etc

- The diet isn't realistic for long-term success

- Can be difficult for many dieters to completely eliminate sweet and starchy foods

- Calories are below that recommended by most health experts for healthy weight loss

✓ **How it works**

This is a five day low-fat, low-calorie, nutritionally-balanced five-day eating plan designed to leave you feeling full while giving you everything you need to stay healthy. The meals in this plan are low fat and low calorie but still packed with vitamins and fibres so you will lose weight without missing out on anything.

✓ **How much weight can I lose?**

A dress size in five days!

✓ How it works

This low-fat, low-calorie diet will ensure you lose weight by eating a high concentration of fruit and vegetable, which floods your system with vitamins and minerals, leaving you feeling healthy and glowing. A typical detox diet involves a period of fasting, followed by a strict diet of fruit, vegetables, fruit juices and water. Sometimes, the meal can also include herbs, teas, supplements, and colon cleanses or enemas.

✓ How much weight can I lose?

It varies from person to person, but you

should feel lighter and more nourished in just 7 days.

✓ **Pros**

- Rest your organs by fasting
- Avoiding dietary sources of heavy metals and POPs
- Stimulate your liver to get rid of toxins
- Promote toxin elimination through faeces, urine, and sweat
- Improve circulation
- Provide your body with healthy nutrients

✓ **Cons**

- Severe calorie restriction
- Can be costly to buy organic food

- Some detox diets may pose the risk of overdosing on supplements, laxatives, diuretics, and even water

- Certain populations include children, adolescents, older adults, those who are malnourished, pregnant or lactating women and people who have blood sugar issues, such as diabetes or an eating disorder.

2.1   Tips for Losing Weight Fast

Losing 5 pounds in one week is a trope you would have seen in different places overtime. And while it's possible for you lose that much and even more in that time period, your success or failure depends on your metabolism and loads of other factors, including physical activity and body composition, all of which are entirely unique to you.

Weight loss essentially revolves around the concept of calories in, calories out: Eat less than you burn and you'll lose weight. And while it's pretty easy to lose water weight quickly on a low-carb diet, it's not recommended. The diet itself can trick you into thinking that this eating style is working — when really, you might gain back what you lost as soon as you eat carbs again. That can feel incredibly dispiriting if you want results that last longer than a week.

If you're looking to speed up weight loss, it's important for you to be mindful of the foods you eat that you don't choose for yourself. For example, swapping sugary beverages for sparkling water or unsweetened tea and coffee is one of the easiest ways to lose weight faster. Other common culprits often come in refined grains like cereals, chips, crackers, and cookies.

Aside noticing where your extra calories come from so you can work towards making better choices in the short and long term, there are a few other tips that you can put into practice beginning right now if you're looking to lose weight fast and effectively.

1. **Eat more vegetables, all of the time**.

Making your meals mostly veggies (at least 50% of anything that you're having) will keep you on the right track to fight off weight gain and prevail.

2. **Build a better breakfast.**

All meals are important, but breakfast is what helps you start your day on the right track. Ideally, your breakfast should fill you up, keep you satisfied, and stave off cravings later in the day. Your goal should be to eat anywhere between 400 and 500 calories for your morning meal, and aim to include a source of lean protein plus filling fat (e.g., eggs, unsweetened Greek yogurt, nuts, or nut butters) and fiber (veggies, fruit, or 100% whole grains). Starting your day with a blood sugar-stabilizing blend of nutrients will help you slim down without stress.

3. **Drink more coffee**.

Start your day with a cup of coffee. Caffeine is a natural diuretic and an excellent source of antioxidants, which protect your cells from damage. According to the Dietary Guidelines for Americans, you can have up to 400 mg of coffee daily.

If you're not a fan of coffee, tea is another very good option. In fact, according to a recent study comparing the metabolic effect of green tea (in extract) with that of a placebo, it was found that the green-tea drinkers burned about 70 additional calories in a 24-hour period.

4. Avoid added sugars.

These include the sugars in cookies, cakes, sugar-sweetened drinks, and other items -- not the sugars that are naturally in fruits, for instance. Sugary foods often have a lot of calories but few nutrients. Aim to spend less than 10% of your daily calories on added sugars.

5. Do strength training.

Straight training can play a sustainable role in your weight loss journey. When you do strength training, you get to build lean muscle tissue which burns more calories — at work or at rest — 24 hours a day, seven days a week. The more lean muscle you have, the faster you'll slim down.

You can start by doing some push-ups or a few squats or lunges three to four times per week. For a rapid improvement, use your free weights to perform simple bicep curls or triceps pulls right in your home or office.

Although women are sometimes hesitant to do weight training because they are afraid they will start to look manly, this is actually a misconception, as women lack the amount of testosterone that men have. Apart from the benefits of building muscle, strength training can also be crucial in increasing your metabolic rate, and preventing diabetes.

6. Eat spicy foods — seriously!

Capsaicin, a compound found in jalapeño and cayenne peppers has been proven to increase the body's release of stress hormones such as adrenaline, which can speed up your ability to burn calories. You're also less likely to wolfed down that plate of spicy spaghetti — and therefore stay more mindful of when you're full.

7. Be choosy about carbs.

You can decide which carbs you eat, and

how much. Ideally, aim for those that are low on the glycemic index (for instance, asparagus is lower on the glycemic index than a potato) or lower in carbs per serving than others. Whole grains are better choices than processed items, because processing removes key nutrients such as fiber, iron, and B vitamins.

8. Cut back on soda

When you drink liquid carbs, like the sugar in soda, your body doesn't register them the same way as, say, a piece of bread, according to a review of studies published in _Current Opinion in Clinical Nutrition & Metabolic Care_. That means, even though you're taking in calories, your fullness cues aren't likely to signal that you're satisfied once you finish off a can. And that can lead to consuming more overall.

Even calorie-free diet soda might keep you from reaching your goals. Though the reason for increased risk for obesity isn't clear, recent research suggests that **artificially sweetened soda could stimulate hunger hormones,** leading people to consume more calories than they need.

9. Get enough sleep

Loads of research has demonstrated that getting less than 7 hours of sleep per night can slow down your metabolism. Plus, when you're awake for longer, you're naturally more likely to snack on midnight munchies. Aim to get enough sleep every night, and you'll be rewarded with an extra edge when it comes to losing weight.

10.   Take a walk before dinner

Although exercising at any time is beneficial, but evening activity may be particularly good for your weight loss agenda because metabolism slows down toward the end of the day. Thirty minutes of aerobic activity before dinner will increase your metabolic rate and keep it high for another two or three hour.

11.   Eat your largest meal at night

Also some <u>research</u> shows that the human body is primed to consume most of its calories during daylight hours. But the lifestyle is problematic for many: After all, when you run out of calories too early to go out to dinner with friends or satisfy a bedtime craving, you're more likely to fall victim to break one "rule" and give up for the rest of the night.

Furthermore, <u>research</u> suggests balanced bedtime meals may also promote steady next-day blood sugar levels, which also helps with appetite regulation.

12.   Never skip a meal.

The truth is skipping meals will not make you lose weight faster. Rather than allowing a hectic day force you to skip a meal, endeavour to stash a piece of fruit and pack of nut butter in your car or purse to avoid going hungry!

Staying long periods of time a day without food does double-duty harm on your healthy eating efforts by both slowing down your metabolism, and priming you for a binge later in the day. Aim to eat three meals and two snacks every day. Ideally, you shouldn't wait longer than three to four hours without eating.

13.   Drink more water

When you skimp on fluids, your body releases an antidiuretic hormone that leads to water retention that could affect the scale. While this sneaky effect is one reason why the scale is a poor measure of body mass loss, you can outsmart it by drinking more—particularly if you fill your glass with water or non-calorie alternatives like unsweetened coffee and tea.

14.   **Manage stress**

Anytime you're stressed, you probably go for food (especially sugary, fatty foods). According to a <u>2007 study on Obesity</u> that quantified chronic stress exposure by looking at cortisol concentrations in more than 2,000 adults' hair, it was found that stress is associated with higher weight. This is why no weight-loss journey is complete without a stress-management tactic.

15.   **Take mineral-rich foods.**

Foods rich in potassium, magnesium, and calcium can help to serve as a counter-balance for sodium. They've also been linked to a whole host of additional health benefits, such as lowering blood pressure, bloat-busting boost, controlling blood sugar, and reducing risk of chronic disease overall. Examples include leafy greens, most "orange" foods (oranges, sweet potatoes, carrots, melon), bananas, low-fat dairy, plus nuts, tomatoes, and cruciferous veggies — especially cauliflower.

16.   Be Accountable

There are many apps that can help you track your calories intake. You can also keep a pen-and-paper food journal of what you ate and when. It is also important to have your family and friends on your side to support your efforts to lose weight. You might also want to join a weight loss group where you can discuss with people who have lost weight in a healthy way. Their encouragement is "contagious," in a good way!

17. Find the eating pattern that works best for you.

If a middle-aged man and woman are both interested in losing weight, the amount of calories a man needs for weight loss are about 1,500 per day (depending on height/weight/level of physical activity), but the woman's calorie needs will be much less — typically about 1,200 calories per day. As a woman, maintaining your weight loss may mean eating less than men in the long term.

18.   Focus on the long game.

It's important to be patient. Studies show that most weight loss plans will typically result in 5% to 10% weight loss within a year if you stick with it. If you aren't seeing results, it is important to talk with your healthcare team as you may need to try a different plan that will suit your lifestyle better.

Whether you follow a diet low in fat, low in carbohydrates or some other diet, make sure meals are balanced and nutritious. Include lean proteins, healthy fats like nuts, olive oil and avocados, limited simple carbs (no sugar, white bread, sweetened drinks) and lots of vitamins and minerals from vegetables and fruit. And if you're above 50, include maintaining adequate calcium and Vitamin D, either from foods or supplements.

19.   Crunch your produce.

Liquid calories aren't as filling as calories from whole fruits and veggies. An orange has about 2.5 g fiber and 47 calories, while 16 oz of orange juice has about 1 g of fiber and 220 calories, so you're better off eating your fruits and veggies rather than juicing them. If you do love juice, try a green one made with naturally low-sugar vegetables like spinach, kale, cucumbers, and celery with a splash of fruit juice for half the calories and a third of the sugar.

20.   Eat More Protein

Protein foods like meat, poultry, seafood, eggs, dairy, and legumes are an important part of a healthy diet, especially when it comes to weight loss. In fact, studies reveal that following a high-protein diet can cut cravings, increase feelings of fullness, and boost metabolism.

21.   Practice Mindful Eating

Mindful eating involves minimizing external distractions during your meal. Try eating slowly and focusing your attention on how your food tastes, looks, smells, and feels. This practice helps promote healthier eating habits and is a powerful tool for increasing weight loss. Eating slowly has been found to enhance feelings of fullness and may lead to significant reductions in daily calorie intake.

22.   Snack Smarter

Selecting healthy, low-calorie snacks is a great way to lose weight and stay on track by minimizing hunger levels between meals. Aim for snacks that are high in protein and fiber to promote fullness and curb cravings.

Whole fruit paired with nut butter, veggies with hummus, or Greek yogurt with nuts are examples of nutritious snacks that can support long-lasting weight loss.

23.   **Squeeze in more steps**

When you're pressed for time and unable to fit in a full workout, squeezing more steps into your day is an easy way to burn extra calories and increase weight loss.

In fact, it's estimated that non-exercise-related activity may account for 50% of the calories your body burns throughout the day.

Taking the stairs instead of the elevator, parking further from the door, or taking a walk during your lunch break are a few simple strategies to bump up your total number of steps and burn more calories.

24. Take a Probiotics Supplement

Probiotics are a type of beneficial bacteria that can be consumed through food or supplements to help support gut health. Studies show that probiotics can promote weight loss by increasing the excretion of fat and altering hormone levels to reduce appetite

25.   Set Attainable Goals

Setting SMART goals can make it easier to reach your weight loss goals while also setting you up for success.

SMART goals should be specific, measurable, achievable, relevant, and time-bound. They should hold you accountable and lay out a plan for how to reach your goals.

For example, instead of simply setting a goal to lose 10 pounds, set a goal to lose 10 pounds in 3 months by keeping a food journal, going to the gym 3 times per week, and adding a serving of vegetables to each mea

MZ International Level 20, AIA Tower,
251A-301 Avenida Comercial De Macau
853 Macau Macau